48
HOURS TO A
HEALTHIER YOU;
Digestive relief you can feel

By: Cori MacLean

Acknowledgements

	I want to thank my husband for all the time he has spend standing by my side, being my strength when I needed a shoulder as I cried, for being my voice of reason when I thought all was lost, and for believing in me as I set out on this new journey.

	I want to thank my little Golden Llama, for giving me a reason to get out of bed each day. For giving my life meaning. To you I will be forever grateful. You taught me the true meaning of never giving up. Thank you for being so understanding and helpful through my hard years. I love you both.

Thank you to my mom and dad, for always being there and for pushing me into being a better me.
	A Special Thanks to Alisha Hudson for helping me when this book was just an idea

Introduction:

	I spent over seven years of my life dealing with various types of abdominal pain. It seemed like no matter what I did, what I ate or how active I was, nothing seemed to help. I found myself in the emergency department multiple times over the years with severe abdominal pains. Due to my young age I was dismissed each time with variations of food poisoning, kidney stones and a "bit" of constipation, but no other investigations were ever warranted. It became harder and harder for me to continue with necessary day to day activities. After years of fighting my own body; dealing with people shaming me for not eating, or being to skinny, I developed depression and anxiety. I couldn't go anywhere or do anything without this excessive sensation following me around. It built up inside until I'd find myself crying on the bathroom floor, honestly believing whatever was happening inside me was going to kill me right there.

In my 30th year, my family and I relocated to a small community north of Canada's capital city. With this relocation came a new family doctor, "Here we go again." was all I could think. "How crazy is this one going to make me feel?" After many discussions and multiple visits, she finally gave me an informal diagnosis of, Irritable Bowel Syndrome (IBS) when I was 32 and with that, an extreme change in diet was required. I was referred to a registered dietitian who could specialize in my new diet and help me understand and transition to a better life.

This is the point that changed my life. As we walk together through this book, it is my hope that you will feel better, stronger and more confident in your everyday life.

Within 48 hours of this newfound diet I experienced multiple symptom reliefs. Within the first week I was feeling better emotionally and physically. This book will walk you through the sciences of the low-FODMAP diet, how to eliminate and reintroduce foods, it also has books, websites and App suggestions. I hope it can sort out a lot of the FODMAP nonsense that comes with the research. This and other books are the first steps in a better life. Join me as we learn about FODMAPS and how you can make changes that best fit your body and specific dietary sensitivities.

Table of contents

Chapter One: My Story
Chapter Two: What is it? Reasons for this diet
Chapter Three: Behind Closed Doors
Chapter Four: High Food vs Low Foods
Chapter Five: Safe Foods & Tips
Chapter Six: The Positives
Chapter Seven: Bringing it all together

Appendix A

References

Chapter 1

My Story

Are you one of the many people in the world that suffers from sporadic abdominal pain? Pain that seems to be unexplainable, coming and going with what seems to be no pattern? Rejected or dismissed at the doctor's office, not knowing what the next step is or where to start? Feeling like your insides are killing you, eating its way through your organs while you lay in agony praying for the pain to stop? Maybe you have been diagnosed with IBS, Crohn's Disease or possibly other intestinal sensitivities like Gluten Intolerance, or Lactose Intolerant. If you feel you have tried everything and nothing helps, it can be a dark and lonely place. Between the pages of this book I will try and hold a little bit of hope for you.

I have spent over seven years of my life
dealing with various types of abdominal pain.
To this day I am still fighting with medical
professionals for testing and other answers I'm
looking for. It seemed like no matter what I did,
what I ate or how active I was, nothing helped.
I thought I was doing all the right things; eating
my favourite fruits and vegetables, walking
regularly, staying active, planning mealtimes
with my family and taking pride in the foods we
ate while still trying to give my body what it
needed. Yet still, almost every day especially
after each meal, I would find myself feeling
bloated, moody, tired and let's not even talk
about how fast the foods could go through my
system and what that would bring while I was
out of the house. I would be feeling cramping
that caused me to think I had to catch my
breath after a marathon, even though I was
sitting still. There is no way I can sugar coat
this, I felt like death was at my door many times
during these episodes or flair ups.

A few different times over the years I
brought myself to the emergency department

at a near-by hospital, in hopes I could catch what ever was going on and get some answers. Due to my young age I was dismissed each time with variations of, food poisoning, kidney stones and "bit" of constipation, but no other investigations were ever warranted. I didn't understand how I could be in this much pain and discomfort and there still be "nothing wrong". All I was told was basically to wait it out and if it got worse to come back in. The reason I was in the emergency department is because it was on the highest scale of pain. Each time I was sent home to wait out the horrific discomfort and prepping myself for yet another disappointing doctor's appointment to try and find some answers.

As the years passed it became harder and harder for me to continue with necessary day to day activities. I did not want to go out and socialize; dealing with the mass amounts of people shaming me for my invisible disorder, accusing me of not taking care of myself, or not eating properly and being to skinny. I knew most people didn't understand, how could they? It was an invisible disorder with what seemed to be no pattern or reason. I just didn't understand, I felt betrayed and attacked by my own body. At this point I had a different doctor assure me I was otherwise healthy, and I shouldn't worry. As you can imagine, I developed depression and anxiety. I closed myself off from going out and did what I did best. I got up each day for my son, pretended everything was ok. With a fake smile and laugh its easy for people to believe you are fine. Dark reality being, I couldn't go anywhere or do anything without this excessive sensation following me around, it would build up inside until I'd find my self crying and disabled with pain and fear. Sometimes it was physical pain, sometimes it was emotional pain, most times it was both. No matter which path it came the darkness came with it.

I didn't want to do anything; I could hardly cook for my family. The anxiety and the anticipated pain would easily cause my hunger to disappear, I would feel immediately sick. I gave my family cheap; microwaveable, extra processed, horrible foods, claiming I ate earlier and wasn't hungry and they could grab something quick. Soon I began to call in to work. One day I unexpectedly walked in with a note saying I couldn't do it anymore and I walked away from so much I cared about. The pain and depression were to much. I spent the following months in bed, crying as my world came crashing down.

I was fighting my own body for basic nutrients and dealing with inconsistent results, desperately trying to find foods that didn't hurt. I found it was easiest to spend days depressed and hiding in my room from the chores building up around me. During the day I would grab a grape here and there and mostly would stuff my face with cookies at night. I was then drugged up on the sleeping medication at night to help cope. I would sleep through the pain and vomit the next morning. It was not pretty, granted maybe cookies were not the best choice but it tasted good and served a purpose.

In the very recent past, I realized my anxiety became a crippling disorder and that I needed deep therapy to help sort out what was happening. My body was changing, and I would become immediately overwhelmed when entering the grocery store, or when I would be invited out to dinner. I would be sure to have a reason to turn down any unexpected outdoor activity or invitation. Everything changed one day when I was walking through the grocery store with my husband. We were doing our regular routine shopping that we have done together every other week for the last 13 years. I was also trying to find something to eat that would not hurt me. I began to feel like everything I looked at had a track record somewhere in my brain that triggered a sense of pain and discomfort. I remember a flash of anger, my pulse and breathing elevated and before I could process the change, I was in a full hyperventilating uncontrollable sob fest in the middle of the store in peak afternoon. How embarrassing, knowing full well everyone is staring and being able to do nothing about it, I couldn't even leave the building; I was stuck in place by a crushing sensation I was sicker than my conscience was aware.

Looking back, I'm thankful that my pre-teen demanded to stay home, and that my husband was by my side. I'm not sure what he could have possibly be thinking during this meltdown of mine, especially since it seemed to come with no more then a second's notice. He just stood there holding me, trying to make sense of my words until the spell dissipated and I was able to function again. This was about a 9-minute episode but seemed to last a lifetime. This point, this was my hardest realization to process; this is where my life was. How could I let this happen? I am a strong independent, well-rounded individual. I teach emotional regulation to toddlers; how could this be. This to me was unacceptable, it was time for some changes.

After years of discussions with my new doctor she finally gave me an informal diagnosis of Irritable Bowel Syndrome (IBS) but was still unwilling to look further into the matter. In the end I was left with doctors' orders of a new extreme diet intervention I had never heard of. FODMAP was the gibberish word that would soon change my life. I was referred to a dietician a few weeks later. He would specialize in my new diet and help me understand and transition to a low-FODMAP lifestyle.

He helped me, now let me try and help you.

Chapter 2

What is it? Reasons for this diet:

By this point you must have more questions than answers, and that's a good thing. I'm happy for the opportunity to introduce a quick guide to a Low-FODMAP lifestyle. Never heard if it? Wondering what all the fuss is about? Curious to know how it is different from other dietary plans that promise results. I have your answers but first, we must start at the foundation, the bottom, the beginning platform on which everything else is built.

FODMAP's- What are they and how they affect the body.
-   FODMAP's are specific short-chain Carbohydrates or sugars that can not be

absorbed or broken down in the small intestine.
- FODMAP sensitivity has symptoms like:
    - ✓ Bloating
    - ✓ Fever
    - ✓ Abdominal pain
    - ✓ Inconsistent bowel movements
    - ✓ Most symptoms that accompany different gastral distresses can be found in this category
- Individuals with IBS, Crohn's Disease, Lactose or Gluten Intolerances, are more likely to benefit from a Low-FODMAP dietary change, but one should always consult a professional before making any drastic changes to make sure this is the right plan for you. Most who have followed this strict diet intervention have noticed results in as little as 24 hours.

FODMAP's is an acronym for *F*ermentable, *O*ligosaccharides, *D*isaccharides, *M*onosaccharides, *A*nd *P*olyols.

Fermentable

Foods that are broken down by the bacteria in your stomach that can cause bloating and gas build up. This term encompasses the other Oligos, Dis, Mono and Polyols. This is the first stage of digestion. As the bacteria eat away at the food, they release different gases into the digestive track.

Oligosaccharides

A variety of foods that fall under two types of carbohydrates: Galacto-oligosaccharides and Fructans. Fructans can be found in such foods as garlic, onion, and wheat. Galacto-oligosaccharides are mostly found in beans.

Disaccharides

Foods that fall under the lactose category. The two sugars found in lactose, glucose and galactose, can not be digested on their own without the help of a third-party enzyme called lactase. If you are a person who is missing or lacking this enzyme you are sure to be lactose intolerant.

Monosaccharides

The carbohydrate called fructose, naturally
found in fruits. This sensitivity can show when
eating foods with the fructose level higher than
the glucose.

And

Finally, an easy thing to remember. Moving
on.

Polyols

This Carbohydrate can be broken down into
Sorbitol and Mannitol. Polyols can be found
naturally in foods and can also be added as an
artificial sweetener to other foods.

Why this diet? Is FODMAP right for me.

"Why not this diet?" is my answer. If you have been struggling for years, what is the harm in trying one more plan? It could change your life. This diet is full of complicated jargon and technical terms that can be hard to sort through. Using the quick guide, you should be able to pick a few foods that you can try and eliminate or add to your diet. If you are very sensitive, this alone should give you some relief. They say seeing is believing, try making a few small adjustments to your day according to the FODMAP dietary plan and see if it helps. I noticed a difference in just a few days. Within a week I was 50% better then I was feeling. After a month, I couldn't believe the outcome. As with all Diet changes, check with your doctor before starting this diet and be sure it is something that you should try.

Chapter 3

Behind closed doors

This part of the book is not going to be for everyone, and It's possibly the hardest thing I have had to write about so far. The point of this chapter is to give the people who have not experienced this torture an insider's view, and If you have been exposed, then you know your not alone. If you are a person who suffers from IBS or other Gastral Intestinal (GI) issues, then there is a good chance you have been diagnosed with anxiety, depression or both. Many mental health issues can be found along side GI problems. Be sure to see your doctor regularly and inform him/her of any changes in your mental or physical health, surround yourself with loved ones, and remember you're not as alone as you feel. There are many resources and people who can help you. I hope this book becomes one of them.

Behind closed doors is where I suffer, behind closed doors is where the pain and grief take root.   When the darkness holds me; I can not escape.
-Cori MacLean. Depression 2019.

Some days are always harder than others, the flair up's can come on within minutes of eating the forbidden foods. They can last for hours or even days depending on the severity of the FODMAP sensitivity.

Hiding from the world
It is not uncommon to find myself naked in the bathroom, contorted into unnatural positions, trying desperately to find relief in any way I can. My clothing feels tight as if they are holding me back and restricting my every movement and breath, I feel hot and begin removing layers, desperately to find a cool spot. My breathing elevates, every muscle tightens, everything begins to hurt, all I want to do is poop, but nothing is happening. I know it

needs to come out, my body knows it must help. Still I can feel it inside trying to move along the intestines. My body now begins contracting, sending shoots of pain down deep into my core, until it makes me scream out in agony, trying to expel this from my body before it becomes toxic. Still nothing happens. I know that if I push to hard it could really hurt something, but my body can't do anything else. Waves and waves of pain and contractions continue to hit, that's when the vomiting began.

When my body felt it couldn't purge using the natural plumbing, it used our built-in alternative root instead. Sitting in the bathroom, while the horrible contractions are trying to empty my bowels, the spasms have now begun to move up my intestines. Now I sit here with my insides, upper abdomen and lower intestines throbbing and contracting, uncontrollably I begin puking. My body falls into this rhythm I can't control or escape. Pressure building up, wave after wave, until I am left sweating, shaking, and feeling I'm about to collapse. Finally, my body gives in, the contracting and shaking slows, the sweating leaves me with such chills I begin to shiver. Slowly I begin to breathe and come back to the present. That's when I would realize... I still didn't poop. This isn't over.

The horror of knowing this is going to happen again sinks in, this is where my depression gets me. I lay crying on the bathroom floor, shaking and exhausted, hating my body with every fiber of my being. This is not the first time; this is not the last. I began to take a stool softener every day, in order to help keep things moving and prevent these episodes from happening. This seemed like a decent solution, until the days after 5 and 6 of me taking it. After that I hit the opposite end of the spectrum, then diarrhea would run my life. I could never find a balance, always flipping back and forth between constipation or diarrhea, and dealing with all the horrors that goes with it. This went on for many years.

When my doctor offered the LOW-FODMAP diet, I was in a very dark place with no direction to go in. I didn't have hopes for this, I felt I was doomed. But, with nothing else to try… I dove in whole heartedly. I am still amaze at the results and how fast relief can be found once you know what to look for.

The 7 Types of stool

When I visited my dietician, I was somewhat overwhelmed with the amount of information I didn't know about my body and the way it was working against the carbohydrates. One of the things that stood out was when he explained to me there are 7 types/classifications of stool. I thought wow really 7? He showed me what was called the Bristol Stool Chart. (see Appendix A) in paper copy. It was listed as such:

Type 1: Separate Hard lumps, like nuts or rocks. -Hard to pass
Type 2: Sausage shaped, but lumpy.
Type 3: Like sausage but with cracks on the surface
Type 4: Like sausage or snake, smooth and soft
Type 5: Soft blobs with clear cut edges

Type 6: Fluffy pieces with ragged edges, a mushy stool

Type 7: watery, no solid pieces. Entirely liquid.

He taught me that our bodies should be between a type 3 and 4. This is a health track. Once I understood this, I found it was easier to tell when a flair up was happening and what to expect out of the episode. I would be able to better predict the severity of the episode, and the how long I would be incapacitated.

Chapter 4

High Foods vs. low Foods:

Since FODMAP's are simple carbohydrates; they simply can not be avoided completely. What we can do, is understand what foods are high in fodmap's and what foods are low. This knowledge can help you make better food choices when eating out and can possibly save you hours of abdominal torture.

Monash University is the founding school behind the development of the FODMAP's, the effects on our bodies and food classification. There is a lot of information that can be found on their website listed in the Next Chapter

Foods with High FODMAPS are the ones you will want to avoid. They are the ones that feel like a cinder block is going threw your intestines as my mom likes to describe it. Here is a list of foods set into grocery categories

<u>Dairy</u>

Food items that have lactose in it are going to work against you, such as:

- Cottage cheese
- Cream cheese
- Ice cream
- Cow's milk
- ricotta
- Yogurt
- Milks made with soybeans
- Sweetened condensed milk.

<u>Grains</u>

Anything that contains:

- Barley
- Rye

- Wheat

Including: most breakfast cereals, biscuits and snack products. These are main ingredients that can be found on labels, always read the ingredients list.

<u>Herbs and Spices</u>

Thankfully except for:
- Onion Powder
- Garlic Powder
- Pre-Mixed seasoning

Most simple and fresh herbs are low-fodmap. Pre-mixes are best to avoid because you can't be sure what is in them or where they were packaged.

<u>Fruits</u>

(This was a list that admittingly made me sad. I love my fruits.)

- Apples & Apple Juice
- Apricots

- Blackberries
- Cherries
- Dried fruits
- Dates
- Grapefruit
- Mangoes
- Nectarines
- Peach's
- Plums
- Pears
- Watermelon

Vegetables

- Artichoke
- Asparagus
- Cauliflower
- Garlic
- Green peas
- Leeks
- Mushrooms
- Onion
- Sugar snap peas
- Shallots

Nuts and Seeds

- Cashews
- Pistachio

Proteins

- Beans
- Soybeans
- Chickpeas
- Most legumes
- Lentils

Beverages

- Carbonated drinks
- Beer
- Chamomile Tea
- Chicory Coffee
- Fennel Tea
- Oolong tea
- Anything with artificial sweeteners or flavouring *read the labels*

*Caffeine is one of the in-betweens. It is known to stimulate the bowels, so it could be good now and again. There is no other relation to the FODMAP's

<u>Condiments and Sweeteners</u>

This section is a little more difficult to define. Condiments and sweeteners are mixes of multiple ingredients. Just like with the spices and herbs, read the labels carefully and when possible use simple ingredients.

You can be sure to fine things you should avoid in most:
- Barbecue sauces
- Salad Dressings
- Yellow Mustard
- Worcestershire Sauce

A good rule of thumb that I was taught to me along my journey is; if it ends in "tol" you should probably avoid it. For example:

- Maltitol
- Mannitol
- Sorbitol
- Xylitol

These can be found in most items you use every day and especially in items that advertise as "sugar free"

Other more natural sweeteners to avoid are:

- Honey
- Agave nectar
- High-fructose corn syrup

If you could avoid some of these foods or better yet, maybe you don't even like most of these foods. If so, that's great, you are that much closer to living a low-fodmap lifestyle.

-Home work-
*Choose one or two items you
purchase on a regular basis. Read
over the ingredients list and nutrition
facts. Can you pick out some things
that match our High-FODMAP list? If
yes, can you think of an alternative
you could make a change to?*

Chapter 5

Safe Foods, tips for success:

I can not stress how important it is to find yourself a few safe foods before you start this food intervention journey. Safe foods include a short list of things you know your body can digest without consequence. Things that are easy to find while you are out, or things that are quick to snack on while at home.

Like with most changes to your eating habits, its not always going to be easy, and there will be days that are harder than others to stay on track. Most diets will recognize it as a cheat day. The unfortunate news in a low-fodmap lifestyle is, there is no room for cheat days. Cheating on this diet will only cause you pain and discomfort. Some days you may find it harder to prepare foods, or maybe the day just got away from you. No matter what your reasons you are human, and it will happen. Try and plan ahead, keep different snacks on hand and explore some foods, find things with big flavour for the days you just want something.

My current safe foods are:
- Chex cinnamon with 2% lactose-free milk
- Eggs, bacon & hash-browns
- Oven roasted carrots
- Chicken and ground beef, if I control what spices are in it.

<u>Tracking</u>

Using tracking sheet are very important when starting a Low-FODMAP plan, it could be one small change that could trigger your sensitivities. The other reason tracking is so important is because you may not be sensitive to all the FODMAP's, maybe just a few. Tracking sheets during the reintroduction stage is essential to expanding your food palette.

Meal Planning

It is important to have a meal plan. Planning and doing the prep work is going to help ensure you are on a successful path to low-fodmap living. If you have mild sensitivity to FODMAP's, just knowing the High and Low foods might be enough to have you feeling better, for some the sensitivity level might be much greater.

If it turns out you are highly sensitive, I suggest talking to your doctor or dietitian about a full FODMAP intervention. The Niagara Health System offers a lot of free resources, PDF's and other valuable information on planning the elimination and reintroduction diet. *always consult with your doctor before making any major changes to your diet*

Books and Things

Sorting through all the information was very over whelming for me. I found it was hard to find all the information I needed. Each section I would search, would lead me to be more and more confused on where to start. To help with this, I have created a list of books, websites and apps that can act as your partner in crime.

Many of these books have full meal and dietary changes already planned. They have everything you need for a full FODMAP lifestyle make over. From the grocery lists, to how to restock your pantry, they also include charts and recipes to help arm you with the best tools for success. Since I am not a dietician, providing a full dietary regiment to follow is out of my comfort zone, but here is my list of favourites that can help.

These are a few of the top resources I found and used when I planned my Intervention.

Books:
- Monash University Low FODMAP diet guide. By: Monash University
- Healthy gut, Flat Stomach. By Danielle Capalino, MSPH, Registered Dietitian.

- Low FODMAP, 28-day Plan. By Rockridge Press
- The FODMAP Elimination Diet. Trial for Irritable Bowel Syndrome. PT1. Niagara Health System
- The Structured FODMAP Food Challenge. PT2. Niagara Health System.

Websites:
- https://www.monashfodmap.com/
- https://www.niagarahealth.on.ca/site/home
- https://stephanieclairmont.com/

Apps: Can be found on both google play and App Store
- Cara, is the main one I use. It has a teal icon with a C that sort of looks like a sliver of moon.

- Monash University Low FODMAP Diet. Is a blue Icon, with an intestine looking symbol and a down arrow.

Chapter 6

The positives: Low FODMAP

Low-FODMAP's are the targets we are aiming for. Just like High-FODMAP's, Lows can be found in all sorts of foods and spices. This list will provide you with a safety net while you explore the LOW-FODMAP lifestyle. Both lists can give you a quick reference when going through the store, or your own cupboard. The first while, it will just be you getting to know the foods you like and what recipes will work in your home.

<u>Dairy</u>
- Almond Milk
- Coconut Milk
- Lactose-free milk

- Soymilk *ONLY if made with soy protein*
- Lactose-free Yogurt
- Brie Cheese
- Feta Cheese
- Cottage cheese
- Swiss
- Parmesan

Grain

- Almond flour
- Amaranth
- Brown Rice
- Corn Flakes
- Oat Bran
- Oats
- Polenta
- Popcorn
- Quinoa
- White Rice
- Some Gluten free bread and pasta *check other ingredients*

Herbs and Spices

- Allspice
- Basil

- Black Pepper
- Cardamom
- Chinese-five spice powder
- Cilantro
- Cinnamon
- Cloves
- Cumin
- Garam Masala
- Lemon Grass
- Nutmeg
- Paprika
- Parsley
- Rosemary
- Saffron
- Tarragon
- Thyme
- Turmeric

<u>Fruit</u>

- Bananas
- Blueberries
- Clementine's
- Cantaloupe
- Grapes
- Guavas
- Honeydew melon

- Kiwi
- Kumquats
- Lemons
- Mandarins
- Oranges
- Plantains
- Pineapple
- Raspberries
- Rhubarb
- Star fruit
- Strawberries

Vegetables

- Bok Choy
- Bell Peppers
- Carrots
- Celery
- Cucumber
- Eggplant
- Endive
- Fennel
- Galangal
- Ginger
- Green Beans
- Squash
- Scallions (Greens)

- Kale
- Leek (Greens)
- Lettuce
- Potato
- Tomato
- Zucchini

Nuts and Seeds

- Fenugreek Seeds
- Fennel seed
- Coriander seeds
- Mustard Seed
- Macadamias
- Peanuts
- Pumpkin Seeds
- Walnuts

Protein

- Beef
- Canned* Chickpeas
- Chicken
- Clams
- Eggs
- Firm tofu
- Fish
- Lamb

- Lobster
- Mussels
- Oysters
- Pork
- Salmon
- Sardines
- Scallops
- Shrimp
- Tempeh
- Tuna
- Turkey

Beverages

- Black Tea
- Coffee
- Green tea
- White Tea

Condiments and Sweeteners

- Dark Chocolate
- Maple Syrup
- Rice Malt Syrup
- Table sugar

chapter 7

Bringing it all together

So now you have the basic knowledge and understanding of a low-fodmap diet and how it can work for you. You should now be able to implement some changes into your everyday and begin feeling better and living a better life.

The steps in a Full Intervention are:

- Elimination Diet
- Strict 28-day regiment
- Planned Reintroduction of foods
- Journal tracking of foods and symptoms
- Learning triggers
- Living a better life

Remember:

- Talk to your Doctor or Registered Dietitian
- Plan your meals
- Have tasty snacks on hand
- Prep and prepare

And most importantly, *you are not alone*. There is help.

This book is not to be taken as certified health advice, talk to your local doctor or dietitian

<u>Recipes</u>

Roasted Carrots
Servs 2.

You will need:
½ pound carrots
1 tablespoon coconut oil
½ teaspoon garam masala or
salt and pepper
Soft brown sugar

Pre heat the oven to 425 degrees Fahrenheit.
Line a baking sheet with tin foil.

Wash and peel carrots. Cut up so that all pieces are about the same size. I like to make carrot sticks (cut in ½ the long way). My son eats them better that way. Warm/Melt the oil. Brush on oil cover carrots completely. To add extra sweetness and guarantee me boy to eat, I will sprinkle brown sugar after the oil to bake in a little sweetness. Then add spices of your choice. Roast in the oven for 20 minutes carrots are done when they are slightly Brown on the edges.

Cinnamon Sweet Potato's
Servs. 2

You will need:
1 tablespoon olive oil, plus more for the
cooking sheet
1 large sweet potato
½ Teaspoon ground Cinnamon

Pre heat the oven to 425 degrees
Fahrenheit. Line a baking sheet with tin foil and
lightly oil foil to prevent sticking.

Wash, peel, and chop sweet
potato into cubs. Toss in a bowl with oil and
coat evenly. Spread out potato's on prepared
baking sheet evenly in a single layer. Sprinkle
with cinnamon. Roast for 30 minutes and check.
When cubes are slightly brown and soft, they
are ready to enjoy.

Chocolate Bread Rolls

Servs 6

You will need:
      200g Rice flour
      100g Corn flour
      1tsp. Baking powder
      4tbs. Lactose free milk.
      4tbs. rapeseed oil
      250g lactose free quark
      2 eggs
      Dark chocolate

Break the dark chocolate up into small pieces. Mix all ingredients in our whole 2 form a dough. Leave the dough to stand for 10 minutes. Pre-heat oven to 350 degrees Fahrenheit. Next shape into small bread rolls. Coat with one egg yolk at your leisure bake the bread rolls in a preheated oven for 15 to 20 minutes.

Thank You

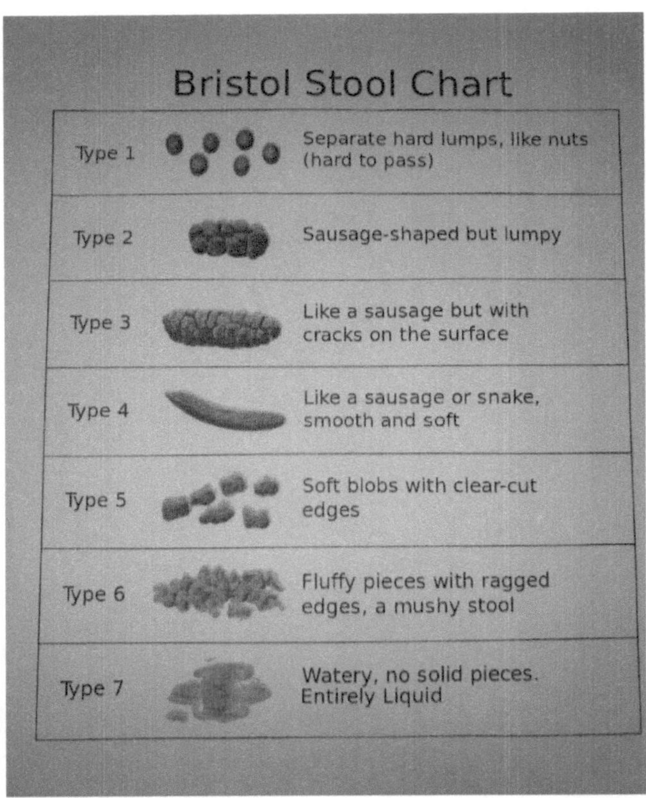

References

D.Capalino (2017). Healthy Gut. Flat Stomach.

Gibson (2017)
https://www.ncbi.nlm.nih.gov/pubmed/28244673

Monash University (2019)
https://www.monashfodmap.com/about-fodmap-and-ibs/high-and-low-fodmap-foods/

Stephanie Clairmont (2019)
https://stephanieclairmont.com/

9 781693 917363